Reinforced Periodontal Instrumentation and Ergonomics
for the
Dental Care Provider

Reinforced Periodontal Instrumentation and Ergonomics
for the
Dental Care Provider

Diane Millar, R.D.H, M.A.

Wolters Kluwer | Lippincott Williams & Wilkins
Health

Philadelphia • Baltimore • New York • London
Buenos Aires • Hong Kong • Sydney • Tokyo

Acquisitions Editor: John Goucher
Managing Editor: Kevin Dietz
Production Editor: Gina Aiello
Production Manager: Caren Erlichman
Design Coordinator: Steve Druding
Compositor: Hearthside Publishing Services
Printer: IMAGO

9 8 7 6 5 4 3 2 1

Library of Congress Cataloging-in-Publication Data
Millar, Diane.
  Reinforced periodontal instrumentation and ergonomics for the dental care provider / Diane Millar.
     p. ; cm.
  ISBN-13: 978-0-7817-9944-7
  ISBN-10: 0-7817-9944-9
  1. Dental instruments and apparatus. 2. Periodontics–Instruments. 3. Human engineering. 4. Dental personnel–Health and hygiene. 5. Dental offices–Safety measures. I. Title.
  [DNLM: 1. Human Engineering–methods. 2. Periodontics–methods. 3. Occupational Diseases–prevention & control. WU 240 M645r 2007]
  RK681.M45 2007
  617.6'32–dc22

                                                                            2007001945

DISCLAIMER

Care has been taken to confirm the accuracy of the information present and to describe generally accepted practices. However, the authors, editors, and publisher are not responsible for errors or omissions or for any consequences from application of the information in this book and make no warranty, expressed or implied, with respect to the currency, completeness, or accuracy of the contents of the publication. Application of this information in a particular situation remains the professional responsibility of the practitioner; the clinical treatments described and recommended may not be considered absolute and universal recommendations.

The authors, editors, and publisher have exerted every effort to ensure that drug selection and dosage set forth in this text are in accordance with the current recommendations and practice at the time of publication. However, in view of ongoing research, changes in government regulations, and the constant flow of information relating to drug therapy and drug reactions, the reader is urged to check the package insert for each drug for any change in indications and dosage and for added warnings and precautions. This is particularly important when the recommended agent is a new or infrequently employed drug.

Some drugs and medical devices presented in this publication have Food and Drug Administration (FDA) clearance for limited use in restricted research settings. It is the responsibility of the health care provider to ascertain the FDA status of each drug or device planned for use in their clinical practice.

To purchase additional copies of this book, call our customer service department at **(800) 638-3030** or fax orders to **(301) 223-2320**. International customers should call **(301) 223-2300**.

Visit Lippincott Williams & Wilkins on the Internet: http://www.lww.com. Lippincott Williams & Wilkins customer service representatives are available from 8:30 AM to 6:00 PM, EST.

PREFACE

Reinforced Periodontal Instrumentation and Ergonomics for the Dental Care Provider was created to address the need for protective ergonomic instrumentation techniques to extend career longevity in a field that has documented evidence of ergonomic disorders. No longer is scaling exclusively about calculus removal. It is about calculus removal and protecting oneself from injury. This book presents new, innovative reinforced instrumentation techniques designed to ensure optimum performance and promote occupational health and career longevity.

Reinforced technique may vary, but essentially the technique utilizes both hands while scaling in order to apply more lateral pressure to the instrument blade and increase control while scaling. Reinforcement also provides more power and improved adaptation which leads to enhanced precision of the instrumentation blade. It is especially pertinent to know reinforced techniques when the student or dental care provider is having difficulty using the one-handed conventional technique while working on a patient that has heavy calculus.

This book is an innovative educational tool that shows, by use of color photographs, the reinforced instrumentation technique in all areas of the mouth. Each instrumentation page explains how to implement protective ergonomic hand, wrist, and arm positions coupled with correct operator positioning. The book emphasizes that dental care providers need not compromise posture to clearly see the working area. It shows the importance of magnification in order to sit in an ergonomically correct position that will allow for more effective scaling techniques. The book also stresses the importance of stretching and exercise to increase muscular endurance and to increase strength and flexibility to help prevent cumulative trauma disorders.

If the dental care provider has a prior injury, this book can be utilized to learn new preventive instrumentation strategies coupled with protective ergonomic positioning skills to help prevent the occurrence of additional work-related injuries. Work-related injuries are discussed in the book along with multiple strategies for prevention.

This book can be beneficial for employers as well as hygienists in private practice to reduce the incident of injury which leads to work-related disability and worker's compensation claims. The claims associated with work-related injuries in dentistry are disruptive, and the costs are significant. Fortunately though, prevention measures can be implemented to reduce work loss, pain, and chronic long-term disability.

The flip chart format of Reinforced Periodontal Instrumentation and Ergonomics for the Dental Care Provider provides a quick-reference, user-friendly interface, allowing for efficient navigation through the various topic sections with detailed pictures and easy-to-understand instructions. The book is organized into 19 chapters:

Chapters 1–6 This section includes the introduction to reinforced instrumentation technique and discusses the advantages of using reinforcement while scaling and guidelines for success. Prevention awareness and protection is the primary focus. A page on strategies to prevent musculoskeletal hand injuries lists suggestions for the student and the dental provider to implement while scaling. The importance of selecting protective ergonomic instrument design is also discussed. Several pages are devoted to stretching for tension reduction, increased range of motion, wellness, and career longevity. The section continues with the benefits of optical magnification loupes to improve visual acuity. The important topic of around-the-clock positioning while scaling, and the advantages of standing versus sitting in order to access difficult areas on the mandibular arch are also discussed.

Chapters 7–17 Step-by-step instruction and guidelines for scaling the maxillary arch using the reinforced technique are depicted in this section. Four instruments, which include the Gracey 11/12, 7/8, 13/14, and 5/6, are demonstrated for the mesial aspect, direct buccal aspect, direct lingual aspect, and anterior aspect. A photo comparison of the most ideal reinforcement technique is next to the conventional technique at the top of the page. The reinforcement technique shows how the non-dominant hand assists and reinforces the dominant hand. In conjunction, many additional reinforcements are shown at the bottom of the instrumentation pages. There are some areas intraorally where additional instrumentation techniques cannot be implemented; therefore, some pages may not have additional reinforcements at the bottom of the page.

Chapters 18–19 These chapters discuss ergonomics and musculoskeletal health in dentistry. Also included is information that pertains to joint hyperlaxity. Many students and dental care providers are unaware that flexible joints can inhibit scaling efficacy and ultimately lead to injury if precautionary scaling techniques are not implemented. Bullet points for protective postural strategies and postural patient positioning, as well as for optimum musculoskeletal health, are listed in this section. The final pages briefly explain work-related hand, arm, and shoulder injuries commonly seen amongst dental care providers coupled with abnormal spinal anatomy from prolonged constrained posture.

I am hopeful that this book will offer the student and the dental care provider new options to scale more efficiently to prevent accidental occupational injuries. Knowledge is power! I truly believe that learning and incorporating new, innovative reinforced scaling techniques will insure protective strategies, peak performance, optimum musculoskeletal health, career satisfaction, and career longevity.

—Diane Millar, RDH, MA

ACKNOWLEDGMENTS

I would like to thank these individuals for offering their precious time, expertise, and encouragement while the book was being developed.

- In memory of Fran Mulvania—writer, author, public relations specialist—who unfortunately passed away three months after the inception of my book. Her belief in me inspired me to move forward with my dream. I will be forever grateful for the time we shared with one another.

- Eula Palmer, my incredible graphic artist, who was instrumental in the design and beauty of this book. Her support and commitment was constant from the beginning. I couldn't have done this book without her.

- Barbara DeMarco Barrett—writer, author, friend—who made helpful suggestions and contributions to all aspects of the book. Her expertise and support is sincerely appreciated.

- Beverly Lovelace, RDH, MS, my right hand throughout the inception and development of this book. I will be forever grateful for her support, knowledge, and friendship.

- Peter Hohenbrink, my photographer, who took many photographs including all the beautiful instrumentation photographs. His talent and expertise is truly incredible and very much appreciated.

- Jen Bierman, Photojenic Photography, who took all of the special-effect exercise photographs. Her creativity and expertise is amazing.

- Elaina Millar, my beautiful daughter and model in all of the instrumentation photos, who devoted many hours in the dental chair. I will be forever thankful for her effort in supporting me.

- Michael Millar, DC, my husband, for his contributions on ergonomics and chiropractic and for his continued support throughout the inception and development of my book.

- Robert London, DDS, Director of Graduate Periodontics at University of Washington—mentor and friend—who encouraged me to lecture on reinforced instrumentation which ultimately inspired me to write this book. I am so thankful for his vision and support.

- Ina Zive, RDH, EdD, retired Dental Hygiene Program Director, Cerritos College—dental hygiene mentor and friend—who devoted many hours reviewing my work and discussing ideas. I am so thankful for her inspiration and support.

- Pat Stewart, RDH, PhD, retired Dental Hygiene Program Director, Cerritos College—dental hygiene mentor and friend—who provided helpful detailed comments and suggestions. Her contribution is truly appreciated.

- Several colleagues, family members, and friends were incredibly generous with their expertise: Brian Killeen, DC; Cindy Litsis, RDH; Denise Jordan, RDH; Linda Laurie; Mark Gibson; Sheryl Cherrison, and Arlene Farinacci.

- John Goucher, acquisitions editor, for his vision and inspiration to have my book published by LWW. I am truly thankful for all of his efforts.

- Kevin Dietz, managing editor, who helped guide and support me while writing the book. I am thankful for all of his recommendations.

- A special thank you to the hygiene faculty and students at Cerritos college for their enthusiasm, support, and encouragement from inception to completion.

—*Diane Millar, RDH, MA*

CONTENTS

CHAPTER 1

Reinforced Instrumentation Technique

einforced instrumentation technique is an advanced protective scaling technique that allows the operator to use both hands while scaling. The reinforcement techniques include:

- Thumb to adjacent thumb reinforcement
- Forefinger to instrument reinforcement
- Thumb to instrument reinforcement

The conventional scaling technique requires the operator to use the mirror for indirect vision. The reinforced scaling technique requires that the operator use direct vision, which allows the nondominant hand to assist the dominant hand while scaling.

Advantages of Using Reinforced Instrumentation Technique

- Enhances the balance of both hands
- Increases control of the instrument blade
- Increases lateral pressure
- Helps to prevent instrument slippage
- Improves scaling efficiency
- Increases power
- Helps to prevent musculoskeletal injuries
- Enhances career longevity by preventing injury
- Encourages the use of larger muscle groups over smaller muscle groups to help prevent repetitive motion injury
- Assists individuals who have hyperlaxity where the thumb and fingers collapse while grasping and activating the instrument
- Helps to decrease hand, wrist and arm pain

Important Factors for Successful Reinforced Instrumentation

- In order for reinforced instrumentation to be successful, proper ergonomic positioning must be employed while instrumenting
- The instrument being held frequently needs to bisect and rest between the thumb and forefinger for more stability and power
- The thumb, if collapsible, needs to be slightly convex or bent
- The thumb on the nondominant hand needs to bridge over to the thumb on the dominant hand for support and assistance
- It is necessary that both hands work together as a unit in order to establish more power ■

CHAPTER 2

Protective Instrumentation Strategies

Suggestions to Prevent Musculoskeletal Hand Injuries

- Wear comfortable, fitted gloves that do not restrict or impinge movement
- Keep fingernails short to be able to fulcrum correctly
- Keep hand, wrist, and arm in a neutral position while scaling
- Use intraoral and extraoral fulcrums with reinforcement of the nondominant hand
- Use direct vision in order to scale with both hands
- Stretch your hands throughout the appointment to help reduce stress and fatigue
- Alternate appointments requiring definitive quadrant scales with maintenance appointments
- Alternate working in areas where there is heavy, tenacious calculus to other areas that require less power and strength
- Shorten the patient's recall interval if lack of home care requires intense scaling at every appointment

Instrument Design and Selection to Help Prevent Injury

- Use rigid shank instruments to reduce repetitive motion
- Use #4 or #6 diameter instrument handles to reduce hand stress and strain
- Use serrated instruments to facilitate instrument grip and control
- Use instruments and hand pieces designed with balanced weight
- Utilize longer-shanked instruments or mini instruments to access deep periodontal pockets
- Maximize the use of ultrasonic scalers to reduce gross deposits and help minimize intense hand scaling
- Maintain blade sharpness to reduce lateral pressure, improve tactile sensitivity, and minimize stress and fatigue ■

CHAPTER 3

Stretching for Wellness and Career Longevity

Most dental professionals do a great deal of sitting while working. Being in a sitting position for long periods of time can cause muscle tension and stiffness. It also leads to weak musculature and restriction of movement in the joints. This can predispose an individual to a musculoskeletal injury, which can reduce career longevity.

Stretching regularly is advantageous for the dental professional. Taking a few minutes to stretch during the day is important for the following reasons:

- Helps prevent muscle strains and sprains

- Reduces tension by increasing blood flow and oxygen to the muscles

- Increases range of motion, which promotes increased flexibility

- Increases coordination, which enhances control of fine motor skills

- Promotes psychological well-being by reducing stress

- Promotes endurance during a stressful day

You can stretch any time and any place. It takes only a few minutes to stretch your back, arms, hands, and shoulders if you are experiencing discomfort from strain. It is of utmost importance to listen to your body and have body awareness when pain is being elicited from lack of mobility, stress, or strain. If you allow yourself to stretch and relax for a couple of minutes during intense moments of discomfort or pain, you will feel better and have more endurance. Your increased level of comfort will also provide a sense of calm and relaxation, which will allow you to feel your best and perform your best in the workplace.

Exercise Outside the Workplace Functional strength training such as Pilates addresses weak core musculature and restriction of movement in the joints that occur from sitting for long periods of time. The Pilates exercises combine a systemic approach to core stabilization of the abdominal muscles, internal and external obliques, erector spinae, and glutes. Core strengthening increases the length in the spine and improves musculoskeletal balance and health.

Flexibility training such as yoga can assist in balancing musculature. Yoga will help stretch, strengthen, and lengthen muscles. Proper flexibility training reduces tight muscles and improves posture, balance, and function. Yoga postures, relaxation, and meditation also reduce stress.

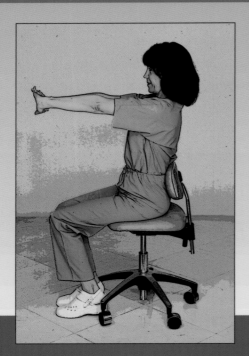

Hand, Wrist, Arm, Shoulder Stretch

Hold 15-20 Seconds Each Arm

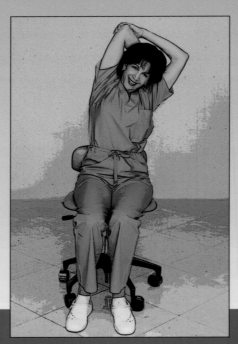

Triceps Stretch

Hold 8-10 Seconds Each Arm

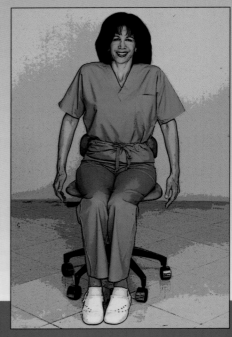

Shoulder Stretch

Hold 5 Seconds
Repeat 3 Times

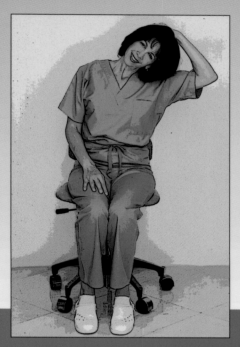

Neck, Upper Back Stretch
Hold 20 Seconds Each Side

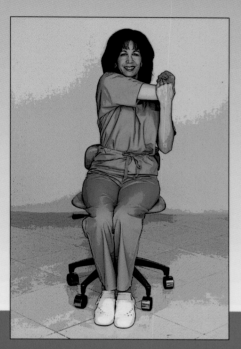

Shoulder, Arm Stretch
Hold 15 Seconds Each Arm

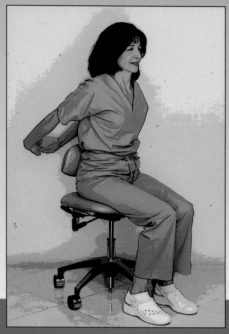

Chest, Shoulder, Arm Stretch
Hold 10-15 Seconds
Repeat 2 Times

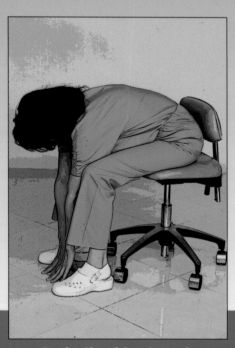

Back, Shoulder Stretch
Hold 10-20 Seconds

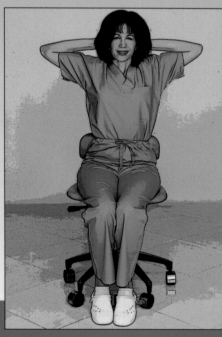

Upper Back, Shoulder Stretch
Hold 5 Seconds
Repeat 2 Times

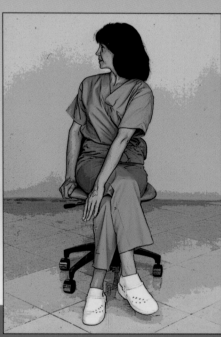

Back, Hip Stretch
Hold 8-10 Seconds Each Side

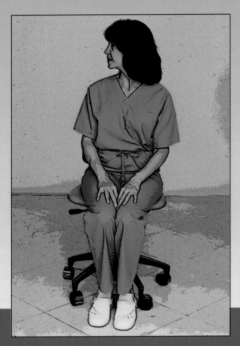

Neck Stretch

Hold 8-10 Seconds Each Side

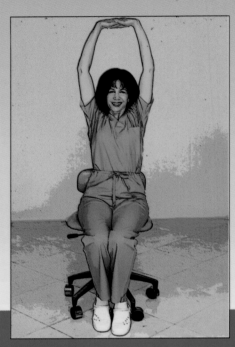

Upper Back, Arm Stretch

Hold 15 Seconds

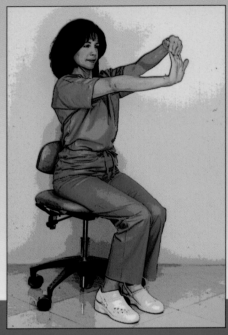

Hand, Wrist, Arm, Shoulder Stretch

Hold 15-20 Seconds Each Arm

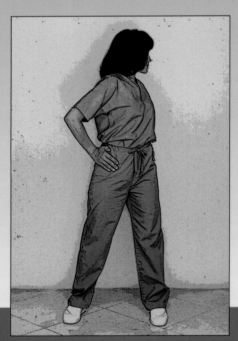

Back, Hip Stretch

Hold 8-10 Seconds Each Side

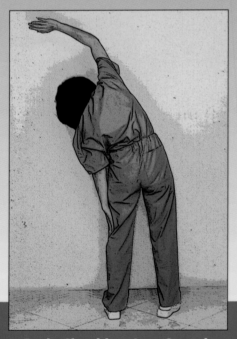

Back, Shoulder, Arm Stretch

Hold 8-10 Seconds Each Side

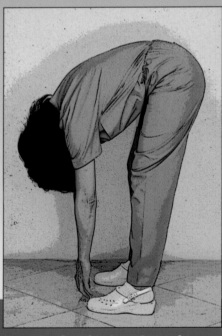

Back, Hip, Leg Stretch

Hold 10-15 Seconds

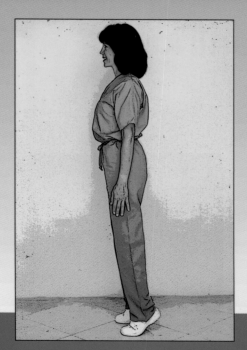

Leg, Foot Stretch
Hold 10-15 Seconds

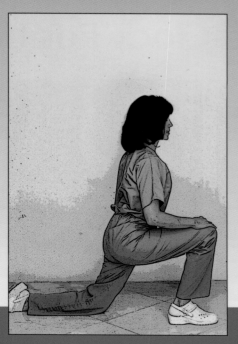

Hip, Leg Stretch
Hold 10 Seconds Each Leg

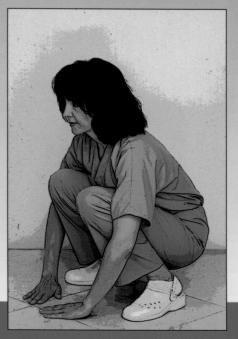

Back, Hip Stretch
Hold 20-30 Seconds ■

CHAPTER 4

Magnification in Dentistry

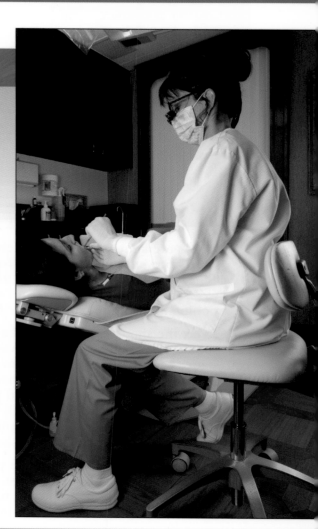

Optical magnification loupes improve visual acuity, ergonomic posture, comfort, and precision in dental procedures. The magnification lenses are measured at an optimal range of distance, which encourages proper sitting posture. The operator's posture is confined to a range determined by the optical depth of field and working distance. If the operator bends too far forward or leans too far back, the object focused upon will appear distorted. Therefore, proper measured fit is critical when using magnification loupes.

Dental hygienists and dentists who do not use magnification loupes often suffer from a multitude of musculoskeletal problems, which include back, neck, and shoulder injuries. These problems often occur due to the need to assume a shorter working distance in order to increase visual acuity.

Many dental hygiene schools are requiring new incoming students to be measured for magnification loupes for the significant benefits of making dentistry more precision oriented, ergonomically safe, and comfortable. ■

CHAPTER 5

Around-the-Clock Positioning

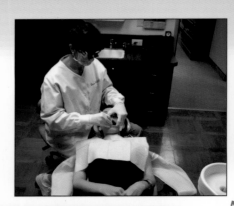
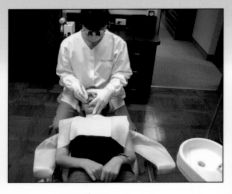
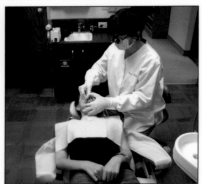
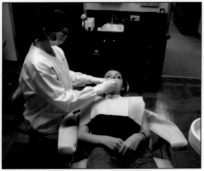
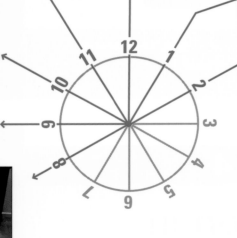
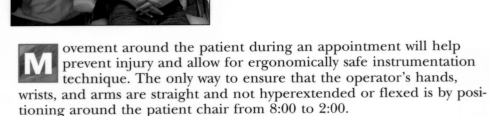

12 11 10 9 8 7 6 5 4 3 2 1

Movement around the patient will help prevent injury and enhance instrumentation technique.

Movement around the patient during an appointment will help prevent injury and allow for ergonomically safe instrumentation technique. The only way to ensure that the operator's hands, wrists, and arms are straight and not hyperextended or flexed is by positioning around the patient chair from 8:00 to 2:00.

Relax the shoulders and keep the spine straight. The operator's hips should be parallel to the floor and balanced over the feet. A runner's stance can be utilized in order to keep the hips angled forward toward the patient's chair. Using a runner's stance and magnification will help assist ergonomic positioning and prevent lateral curvature of the spine while scaling. This technique will assist the operator to sit in a forward position facing the patient. Keeping the spine as erect and straight as possible will minimize musculoskeletal injuries.

It is also important to adjust the patient's head in a position that encourages a straight hand, wrist, and arm position while using instruments. This position, according to biomechanical statistics, is the most protected position for the wrist in order to prevent injury. ■

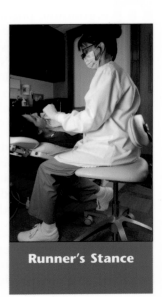

Runner's Stance

CHAPTER 6

Standing when Scaling the Mandibular Arch

Standing in the place of sitting is beneficial during the course of an appointment, especially when working on the mandibular arch and there is difficulty accessing the areas to be scaled.

While standing, the operator will use larger muscle groups in the upper torso and arms when scaling. The use of these muscles provides additional strength, power, and control to remove calculus.

Advantages of Standing when Scaling

- Enhances access intraorally and increases operator visibility while working on the mandibular arch

- Encourages operator movement from sitting in a static position for prolonged periods of time

- Relieves stress and strain on the back by decreasing the intervertebral disc pressure from approximately 220 pounds while sitting to approximately 110 pounds while standing

- Promotes increased cardiovascular blood flow throughout the body

- Allows the operator to stabilize and balance over both hips and feet around the entire chair when scaling on the mandibular arch ■

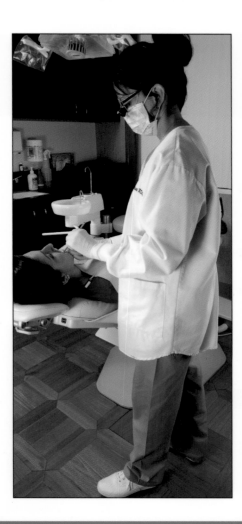
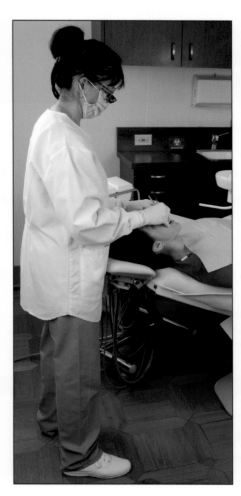
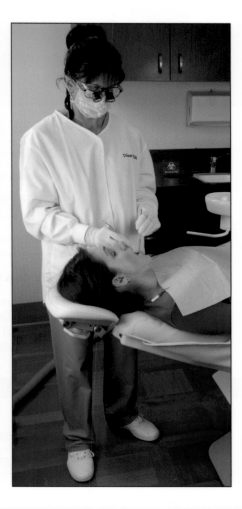

CHAPTER 7

Maxillary Arch, Right Posterior/ Buccal Aspect

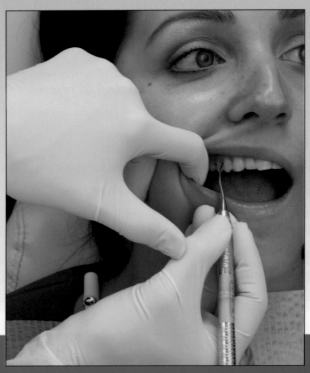

Reinforcement Technique

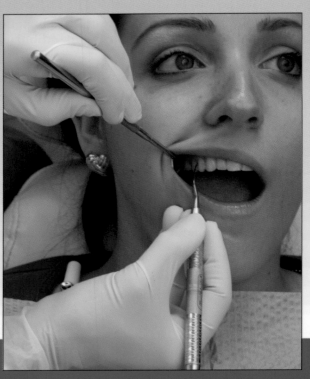

Conventional Technique

Buccal Aspect, Mesial Surfaces

- The **Gracey Curet 11/12** is shown

- **Optional instruments:** 5/6 curet for bicuspids, 15/16 curet for molars

- **Working hand:** Extraoral fulcrum palm up with back of fingers resting against right side of patient's jaw

- **Reinforcement hand:** Left forefinger gently retracts patient's cheek while remaining fingers rest against patient's cheek and jaw

- **Left thumb to right thumb bridging** for reinforcement

- **Technique:** Vertical pull strokes using both hands while utilizing hands and arms as a unit to obtain additional stroke power, lateral pressure, guidance, and stability

Additional Reinforcements

Thumb on shank:

- Extraoral fulcrum: Left forefinger gently retracts patient's cheek

- Left thumb on shank or instrument handle applying lateral pressure

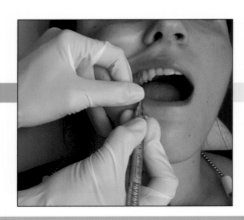

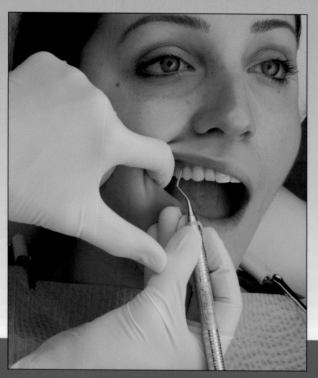

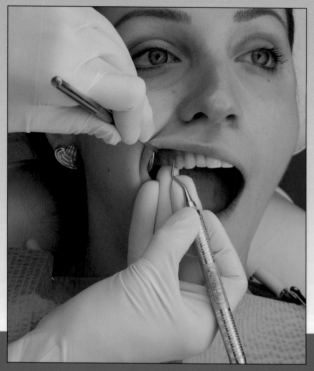

Reinforcement Technique

Conventional Technique

Buccal Aspect, Direct Buccal Surfaces

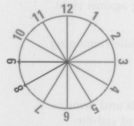

Operator Position:
8:00 - 9:00

Patient Position:
Supine

(Right-handed operator shown)

- The **Gracey Curet 7/8** is shown

- **Optional instrument:** 11/12 curet

- **Working hand:** Extraoral fulcrum palm up with back of fingers resting against right side of patient's jaw

- **Reinforcement hand:** Left forefinger gently retracts patient's cheek while remaining fingers rest against patient's cheek and jaw

- **Left thumb to right thumb bridging** for reinforcement

- **Technique:** Overlapping diagonal and/or horizontal pull strokes using both hands and arms as a unit to obtain additional stroke power, lateral pressure, guidance, and stability

Additional Reinforcements

Thumb on shank:

- Extraoral fulcrum: Left forefinger gently retracts patient's cheek

- Left thumb on shank or instrument handle applying lateral pressure

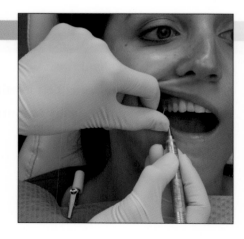

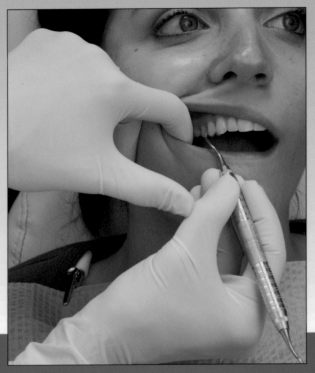

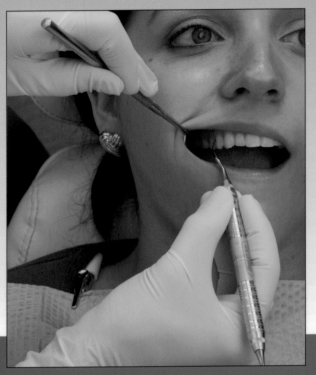

Reinforcement Technique

Conventional Technique

Buccal Aspect, Distal Surfaces

Operator Position:
8:00 - 9:00

Patient Position:
Supine

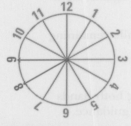

(Right-handed operator shown)

- The **Gracey Curet 13/14** is shown

- **Optional instrument:** 17/18 curet for molars

- **Working hand:** Extraoral fulcrum palm up with back of fingers resting against right side of patient's jaw

- **Reinforcement hand:** Left forefinger gently retracts patient's cheek while remaining fingers rest against patient's cheek and jaw

- **Left thumb to right thumb bridging** for reinforcement

- **Technique:** Vertical pull strokes using both hands while utilizing hands and arms as a unit to obtain additional stroke power, lateral pressure, guidance, and stability

Additional Reinforcements

Thumb on shank:

- Extraoral fulcrum: Left forefinger gently retracts patient's cheek

- Left thumb on shank or instrument handle applying lateral pressure ■

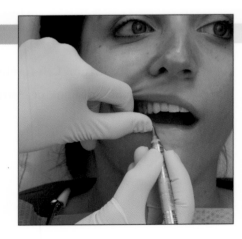

CHAPTER 8

Maxillary Arch, Right Posterior/ Lingual Aspect

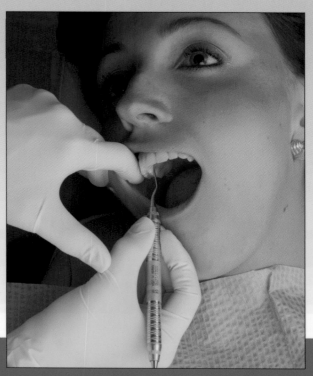

Reinforcement Technique

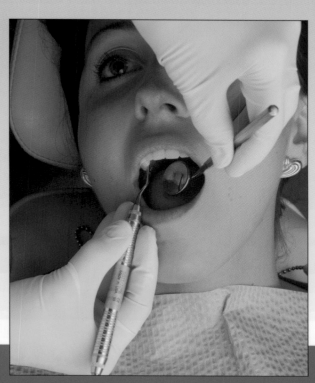

Conventional Technique

Operator Position:
8:00 - 9:00

Patient Position:
Supine

(Right-handed operator shown)

Lingual Aspect, Mesial Surfaces

- The **Gracey Curet 11/12** is shown

- **Optional instruments:** 5/6 curet for bicuspids, 15/16 curet for molars

- **Working hand**: Extraoral fulcrum with back of fingers and hand resting against patient's jaw and chin

- **Reinforcement hand**: Left forefinger positioned in the vestibule of cheek while back side of remaining fingers presses against patient's cheek and jaw

- **Left thumb to right thumb bridging** for reinforcement

- **Technique**: Vertical pull strokes using both hands while utilizing hands and arms as a unit to obtain additional stroke power, lateral pressure, guidance, and stability

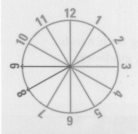

Additional Reinforcements

Thumb on shank:

- Extraoral fulcrum: Left forefinger positioned in the vestibule of cheek; left thumb on shank or instrument handle applying lateral pressure

Pinching shank:

- Extraoral fulcrum: Left forefinger and thumb pinch shank for additional reinforcement and stability.

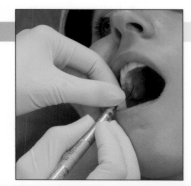

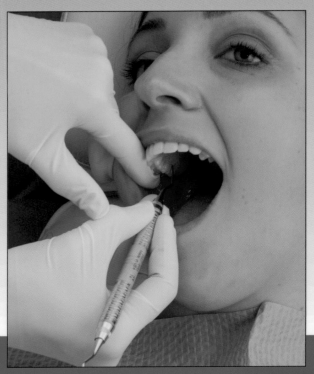

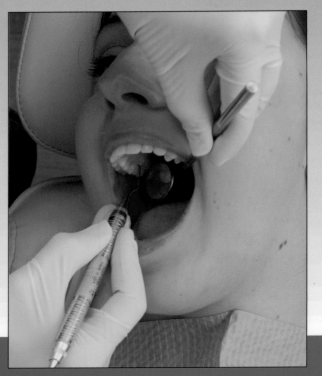

Reinforcement Technique

Conventional Technique

Lingual Aspect, Direct Lingual Surfaces

- The **Gracey Curet 7/8** is shown

- **Optional instrument:** 11/12 curet

- **Working hand:** Extraoral fulcrum with back of fingers and hand resting against patient's jaw and chin

- **Reinforcement hand:** Left forefinger positioned in the vestibule of cheek while back side of remaining fingers presses against patient's cheek and jaw

- **Left thumb to right thumb bridging** for reinforcement

- **Technique:** Overlapping diagonal and/or horizontal pull strokes using both hands and arms as a unit to obtain additional stroke power, lateral pressure, guidance, and stability

Additional Reinforcements

Thumb behind shank:

- Extraoral fulcrum: Left forefinger positioned in the vestibule of cheek while left thumb guides lower end of shank

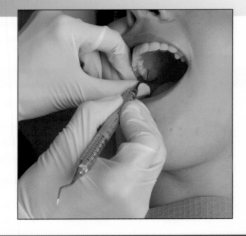

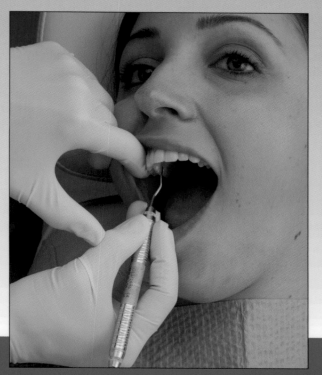

Reinforcement Technique

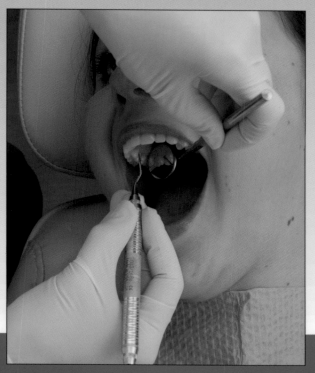

Conventional Technique

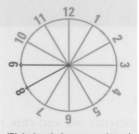
Lingual Aspect, Distal Surfaces

- The **Gracey Curet 13/14** is shown

- **Optional instrument:** 17/18 curet for molars

- **Working hand:** Extraoral fulcrum with back of fingers and hand resting against patient's jaw and chin

- **Reinforcement hand:** Left forefinger positioned in vestibule of cheek while back side of remaining fingers presses against patient's cheek and jaw

- **Left thumb to right thumb bridging** for reinforcement

- **Technique:** Vertical pull strokes using both hands and arms as a unit to obtain additional stroke power, lateral pressure, guidance, and stability

Additional Resources

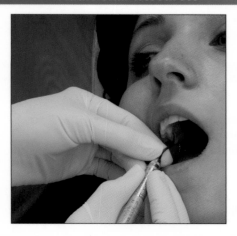

Pinching shank:

- Extraoral fulcrum: Left forefinger and thumb pinch shank for additional reinforcement and control

Index finger behind shank:

- Extraoral fulcrum: Left forefinger gently supports and guides the back of the shank. The remaining back of fingers rests against patient's cheek and jaw for support. ■

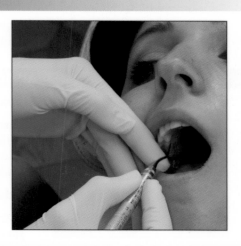

CHAPTER 9

Maxillary Arch, Left Posterior/ Buccal Aspect

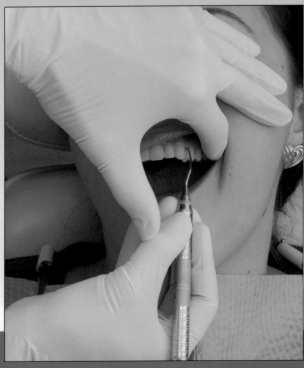

Reinforcement Technique

Conventional Technique

Operator Position:
8:00 - 9:00

Patient Position:
Supine

(Right-handed operator shown)

Buccal Aspect, Mesial Surfaces

- The **Gracey Curet** 11/12 is shown

- **Optional instruments:** 5/6 curet for bicuspids, 15/16 curet for molars

- **Working hand:** Extraoral fulcrum with back of fingers resting against patient's jaw and chin

- **Reinforcement hand:** Left forefinger positioned in the vestibule retracting patient's left cheek while remaining fingers rest on patient's cheek

- **Left thumb to right thumb bridging** for reinforcement

- **Technique:** Vertical pull strokes using both hands while utilizing hands and arms as a unit to obtain additional stroke power, lateral pressure, guidance, and stability

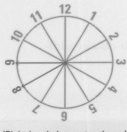

Additional Reinforcements

Index finger on shank:

- Extraoral fulcrum: Back of left forefinger gently retracts patient's cheek while applying pressure on instrument shank. Left thumb fulcrums intraoral on anterior teeth while remaining fingers rest on patient's cheek.

Pinching shank:

- Extraoral fulcrum: Left forefinger and thumb pinch shank for additional reinforcement and control

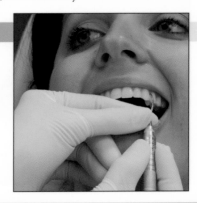

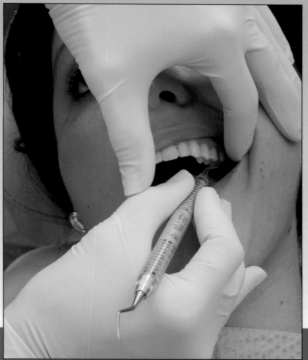

Reinforcement Technique

Conventional Technique

| Operator Position: |
| 8:00 - 9:00 |
| **Patient Position:** |
| Supine |

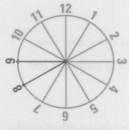

(Right-handed operator shown)

Buccal Aspect, Direct Buccal Surfaces

- The **Gracey Curet** 7/8 is shown

- **Optional instrument:** 11/12 curet

- **Working hand:** Extraoral fulcrum with fingers supported against patient's jaw and chin

- **Reinforcement hand:** Left forefinger positioned in vestibule retracting patient's left cheek while remaining fingers rest on patient's cheek

- **Left thumb to right thumb bridging** for reinforcement

- **Technique:** Overlapping diagonal and/or horizontal pull strokes using both hands and arms as a unit to obtain additional stroke power, lateral pressure, guidance, and stability

Additional Reinforcements

Index finger on shank:

- Extraoral fulcrum: Back of forefinger gently retracts patient's cheek while applying pressure on instrument shank

- Left thumb to right thumb bridging

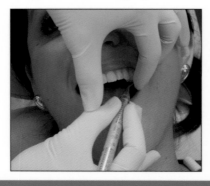

Pinching shank:

- Extraoral fulcrum: Left forefinger and thumb pinch shank for additional reinforcement and control

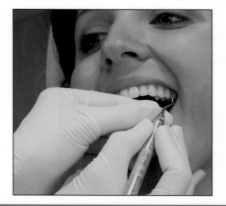

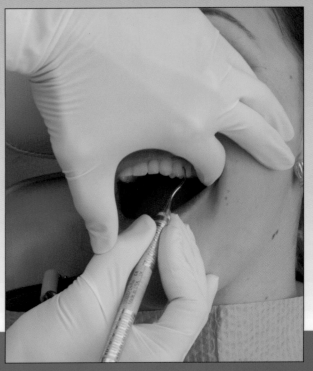

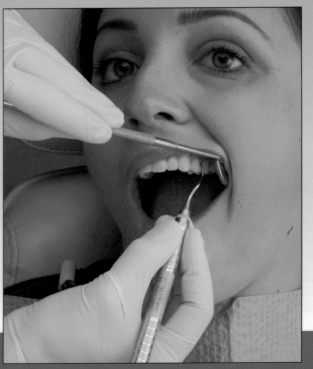

Reinforcement Technique

Conventional Technique

Operator Position:
8:00 - 9:00

Patient Position:
Supine

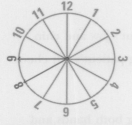

(Right-handed operator shown)

Buccal Aspect, Distal Surfaces

- The **Gracey Curet** 13/14 is shown.

- **Optional instrument**: 17/18 curet for molars

- **Working hand**: Extraoral fulcrum with fingers supported against patient's jaw and chin

- **Reinforcement hand**: Left forefinger positioned in the vestibule retracting patient's left cheek while remaining fingers rest on patient's cheek

- **Left thumb to right thumb bridging** for reinforcement

- **Technique**: Vertical pull strokes using both hands and arms as a unit to obtain additional stroke power, lateral pressure, guidance, and stability

Additional Reinforcements

Pinching shank:

- Extraoral fulcrum: Left forefinger and thumb pinch shank for additional reinforcement and control

Index Finger on shank:

- Extraoral fulcrum: Back of left forefinger gently retracts patient's cheek while applying pressure on instrument shank. Left thumb fulcrums intraoral on anterior teeth while remaining fingers rest on patient's cheek ■

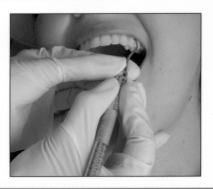

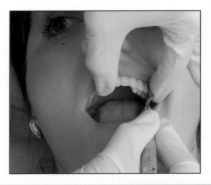

CHAPTER 10

Maxillary Arch, Left Posterior/ Lingual Aspect

Operator Position:
8:00 - 9:00

Patient Position:
Supine

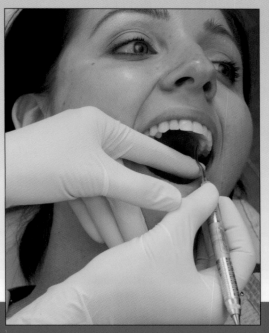

(Right-handed operator shown)

Reinforcement Technique   **Conventional Technique**

Lingual Aspect, Mesial Surfaces

- The **Gracey Curet 11/12** is shown

- **Optional instruments:** 5/6 curet for bicuspids, 15/16 curet for molars

- **Working hand**: Extraoral fulcrum palm up with back of fingers resting against patient's jaw and chin

- **Reinforcement hand:** Left forefinger gently retracts patient's cheek and depresses tongue simultaneously while remaining backs of fingers are bent and supported on patient's cheek and jaw

- **Left thumb to right thumb bridging** for reinforcement

- **Technique:** Vertical pull strokes using both hands while utilizing hands and arms as a unit to obtain additional stroke power, lateral pressure, guidance, and stability

Additional Reinforcements

Index finger behind shank:

- Extraoral fulcrum: Left forefinger gently retracts right cheek while supporting the back of the shank

- Left thumb to right thumb bridging

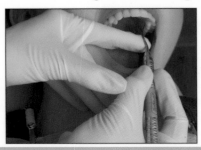

Pinching shank:

- Extraoral fulcrum: Left forefinger gently retracts right cheek while pinching instrument with thumb. Back of hand and remaining back of fingers rest against patient's cheek and jaw for support.

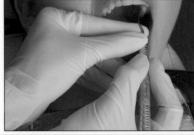

Index finger on shank:

- Extraoral fulcrum: Left forefinger gently retracts right cheek while applying pressure on instrument shank

- Left thumb to right thumb bridging

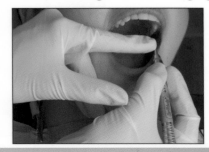

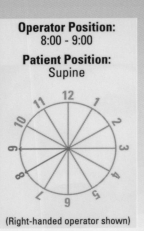
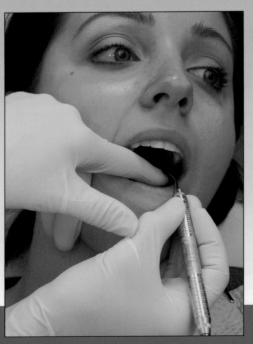

Reinforcement Technique

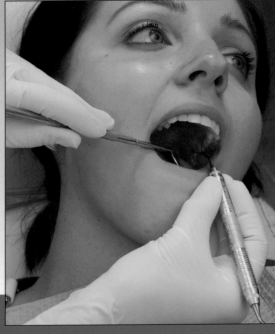

Conventional Technique

Lingual Aspect, Direct Lingual Surfaces

- The **Gracey Curet 7/8** is shown

- **Optional instrument:** 11/12 curet

- **Working hand:** Extraoral fulcrum palm up with back of fingers resting against patient's jaw and chin

- **Reinforcement hand:** Left forefinger gently retracts patient's cheek and depresses tongue simultaneously while remaining backs of fingers are bent and supported on patient's cheek and jaw

- **Left thumb to right thumb bridging** for reinforcement

- **Technique:** Overlapping diagonal and/or horizontal pull strokes using both hands and arms as a unit to obtain additional stroke power, lateral pressure, guidance, and stability

Additional Reinforcements

Pinching shank:

- Extraoral fulcrum: Left forefinger gently retracts right cheek while pinching instrument with thumb and index finger. Back of hand and remaining back of fingers rest against patient's cheek and jaw for support.

Index finger on shank:

- Extraoral fulcrum: Left forefinger gently retracts right cheek while applying pressure on instrument shank

- Left thumb to right thumb bridging

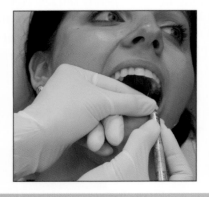

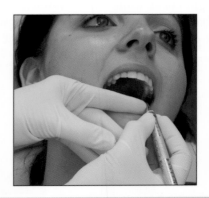

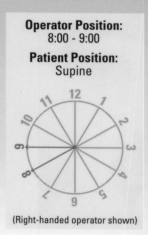

(Right-handed operator shown)

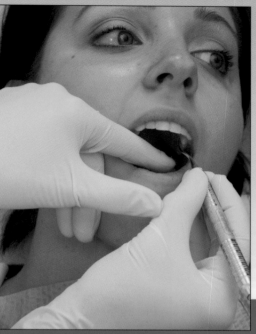

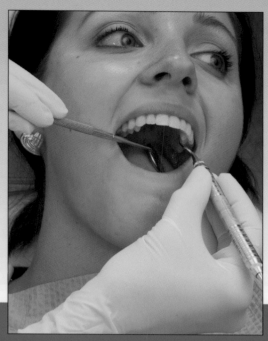

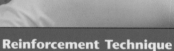

Reinforcement Technique   **Conventional Technique**

Lingual Aspect, Distal Surfaces

- The **Gracey Curet 13/14** is shown

- **Optional instrument:** 17/18 curet for molars

- **Working hand:** Extraoral fulcrum palm up with back of fingers resting against patient's jaw and chin

- **Reinforcement hand:** Left forefinger gently retracts patient's cheek and depresses tongue simultaneously while remaining backs of fingers are bent and supported on patient's cheek and jaw

- **Left thumb to right thumb bridging** for reinforcement

- **Technique:** Vertical pull strokes using both hands and arms as a unit to obtain additional stroke power, lateral pressure, guidance, and stability

Additional Reinforcements

Index finger behind shank:

- Extraoral fulcrum: Left forefinger gently retracts right cheek while supporting the back of the shank

- Left thumb to right thumb bridging

Pinching shank:

- Extraoral fulcrum: Left forefinger gently retracts right cheek while pinching instrument with thumb. Back of hand and remaining back of fingers rest against patient's cheek and jaw for support. ■

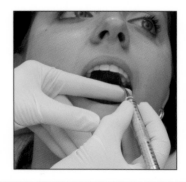

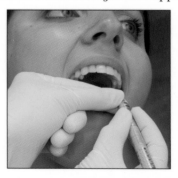

CHAPTER 11

Maxillary Arch, Anterior/Facial Aspect

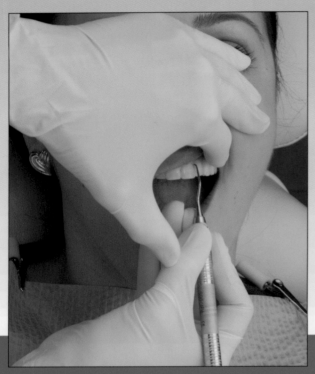

Reinforcement Technique

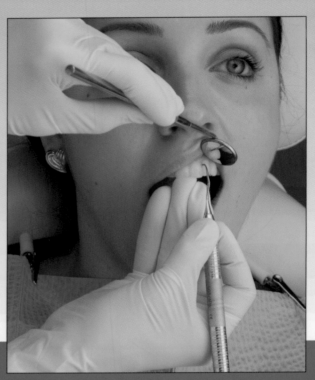

Conventional Technique

Operator Position:
9:00 - 10:00

Patient Position:
Supine

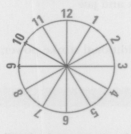

(Right-handed operator shown)

Facial Aspect, Mesial Surfaces

- The **Gracey Curet 5/6** is shown

- **Optional instruments:** 1/2, 7/8, 11/12 curets

- **Working hand:** Extraoral fulcrum palm up with back of fingers resting against patient's jaw and chin

- **Reinforcement hand:** Left forefinger retracts upper lip and rests on maxillary teeth while remaining fingers are stabilized slightly on patient's cheek

- **Left thumb to right thumb bridging** for reinforcement

- **Technique:** Vertical pull strokes using both hands and arms as a unit to obtain additional stroke power, lateral pressure, guidance, and stability

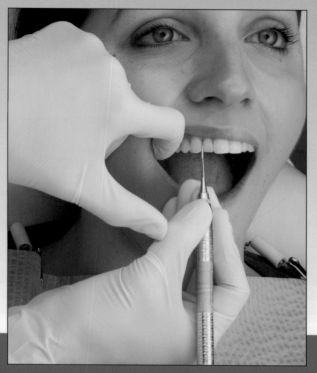

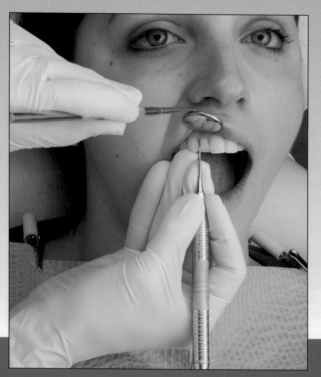

Reinforcement Technique

Conventional Technique

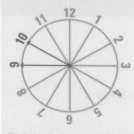
Facial Aspect, Distal Surfaces

- The **Gracey Curet 5/6** is shown

- **Optional instruments:** 1/2, 7/8, 11/12 curets

- **Working hand:** Extraoral fulcrum palm up with back of fingers resting against patient's jaw and chin

- **Reinforcement hand:** Left forefinger retracts upper lip and rests on maxillary teeth while remaining fingers are stabilized slightly on patient's cheek

- **Left thumb to right thumb bridging** for reinforcement

- **Technique:** Vertical pull strokes using both hands and arms as a unit to obtain additional stroke power, lateral pressure, guidance, and stability ■

CHAPTER 12

Mandibular Arch, Right Posterior/ Buccal Aspect

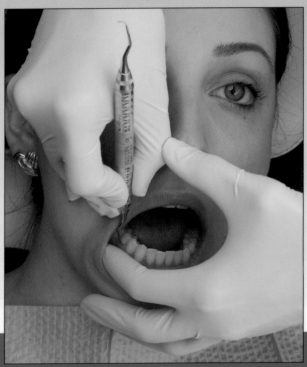

Reinforcement Technique

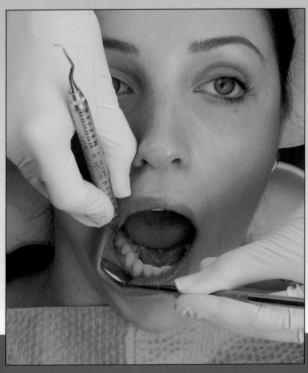

Conventional Technique

Operator Position:
12:00 - 2:00

Patient Position:
Supine

(Right-handed operator shown)

Buccal Aspect, Mesial Surfaces

- The **Gracey Curet 11/12** is shown

- **Optional instruments:** 5/6 curet for bicuspids; 15/16 curet for molars

- **Working hand:** Extraoral fulcrum rests on patient's cheek

- **Reinforcement hand:** Left forefinger retracts lip and rests in vestibule while remaining fingers cup the chin and jaw for stability

- **Left thumb to right thumb bridging** for reinforcement

- **Technique:** Vertical pull strokes using both hands while utilizing hands and arms as a unit to obtain additional stroke power, lateral pressure, guidance, and stability

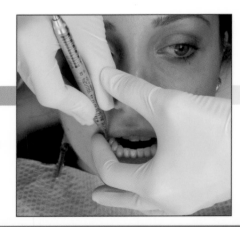

Additional Reinforcements

Index finger on shank:

- Extraoral fulcrum: Left forefinger gently retracts patient's lip and applies pressure on shank of instrument

- Left thumb to right thumb bridging

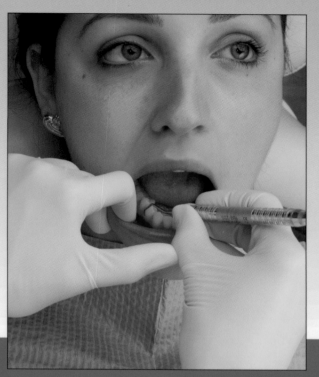

Reinforcement Technique

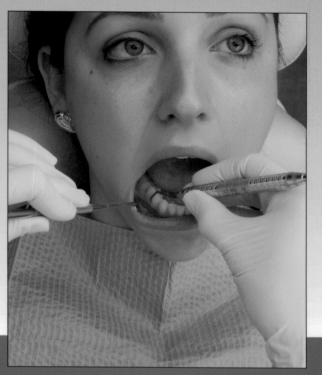

Conventional Technique

Buccal Aspect, Direct Buccal Surfaces

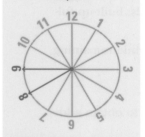

Operator Position:
8:00 - 9:00

Patient Position:
Supine

(Right-handed operator shown)

- The **Gracey Curet** 7/8 is shown

- **Optional instrument:** 11/12 curet

- **Working hand:** Extraoral/intraoral fulcrum with fingers resting on facial aspect of patient's lower anterior teeth and on chin

- **Reinforcement hand:** Left forefinger gently retracts right cheek while remaining back side of fingers rests against patient's cheek and jaw

- **Left thumb to right thumb bridging** for reinforcement

- **Technique:** Overlapping diagonal and/or horizontal pull strokes using both hands and arms as a unit to obtain additional stroke power, lateral pressure, guidance, and stability

Additional Reinforcement

Thumb on shank:

- Extraoral/intraoral fulcrum: Left forefinger gently retracts right cheek while thumb presses on instrument shank

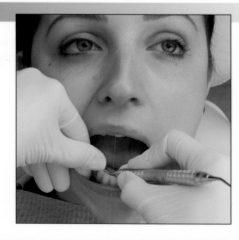

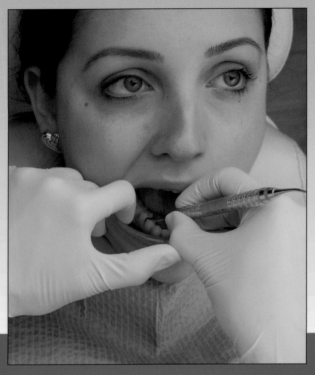

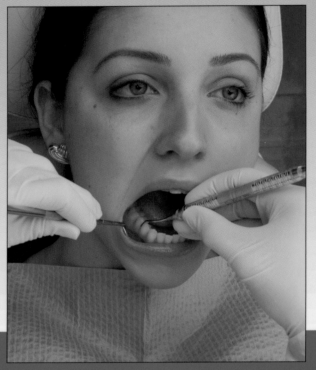

Reinforcement Technique

Conventional Technique

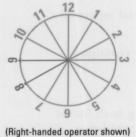

(Right-handed operator shown)

Buccal Aspect, Distal Surfaces

- The **Gracey Curet 13/14** is shown

- **Optional instrument:** 17/18 curet for molars

- **Working hand:** Intraoral fulcrum on mandibular anteriors or bicuspids; built-up fulcrum necessary for parallel shank

- **Reinforcement hand:** Left forefinger gently retracts patient's cheek while remaining fingers and hand rest against patient's cheek and jaw

- **Left thumb to right thumb bridging** for reinforcement

- **Technique:** Vertical pull strokes using both hands and arms as a unit to obtain additional stroke power, lateral pressure, guidance, and stability

Additional Reinforcements

Index finger on shank:

- Intraoral fulcrum: Left forefinger gently retracts patient's cheek and applies pressure on shank of instrument ■

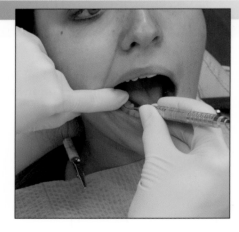

CHAPTER 13

Mandibular Arch, Right Posterior/ Lingual Aspect

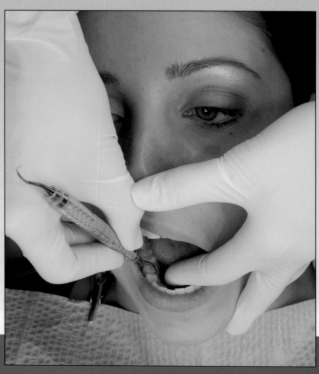

Reinforcement Technique

Conventional Technique

Operator Position:
12:00 - 1:00

Patient Position:
Supine

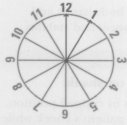

(Right-handed operator shown)

Lingual Aspect, Mesial Surfaces

- The **Gracey Curet 11/12** is shown

- **Optional instrument:** 5/6 curet for bicuspids; 15/16 curet for molars

- **Working hand:** Extraoral fulcrum with fingers stabilized on patient's cheek and jaw

- **Reinforcement hand:** Left forefinger gently retracts tongue while remaining fingers support patient's lower jaw

- **Left thumb to right thumb bridging** for reinforcement

- **Technique:** Vertical pull strokes using both hands while utilizing hands and arms as a unit to obtain additional stroke power, lateral pressure, guidance, and stability

Additional Reinforcements

Index finger on shank:

- Extraoral fulcrum: Left forefinger applies pressure on shank of instrument

- Left thumb to right thumb bridging for reinforcement

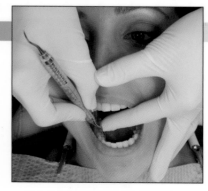

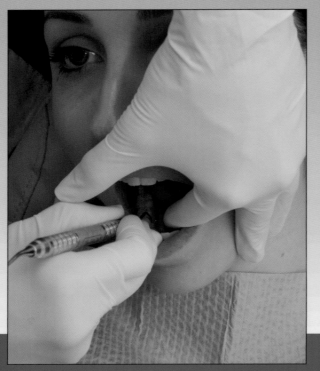

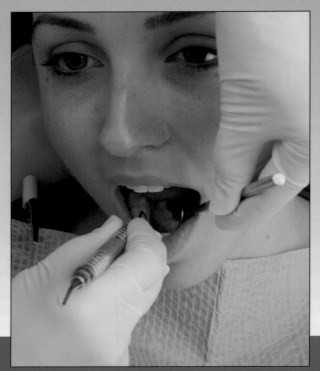

Reinforcement Technique

Conventional Technique

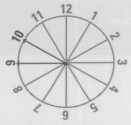
Lingual Aspect, Direct Lingual Surfaces

- The **Gracey Curet 7/8** is shown

- **Optional instrument:** 11/12 curet

- **Working hand:** Built-up intraoral fulcrum close to work site

- **Reinforcement hand:** Left forefinger gently retracts patient's tongue and cheek while remaining fingers press against patient's cheek and jaw

- **Left thumb to right thumb bridging** for reinforcement

- **Technique:** Overlapping diagonal and/or horizontal pull strokes using both hands and arms as a unit to obtain additional stroke power, lateral pressure, guidance, and stability

Additional Reinforcements

Index finger on shank:

- Intraoral fulcrum: Left forefinger gently retracts patient's cheek while applying pressure on instrument shank

- Left thumb to right thumb bridging for reinforcement

Cupping hands, index finger on shank:

- Intraoral fulcrum: Both hands in cupped position. Left forefinger gently retracts patient's cheek while pressing on instrument shank

- Both thumbs pressed together for reinforcement.

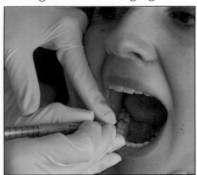

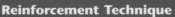

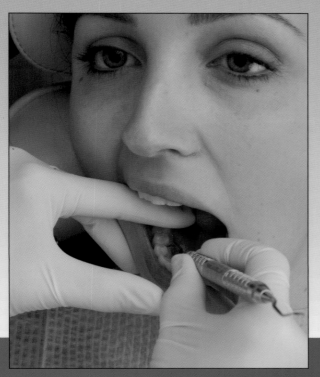

Reinforcement Technique

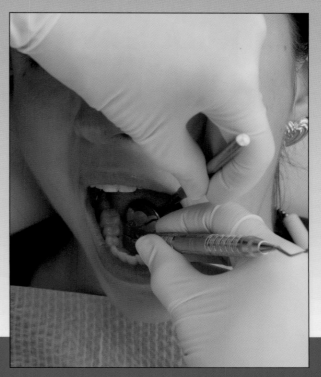

Conventional Technique

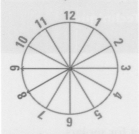

Operator Position:
8:00 - 9:00

Patient Position:
Supine

(Right-handed operator shown)

Lingual Aspect, Distal Surfaces

- The **Gracey Curet 13/14** is shown

- **Optional instrument:** 17/18 curet for molars

- **Working hand:** Built-up intraoral fulcrum close to work site

- **Reinforcement hand:** Left forefinger gently retracts patient's cheek while back side of remaining fingers press against patient's cheek and jaw

- **Left thumb to right thumb bridging** for reinforcement

- **Technique:** Vertical pull strokes using both hands and arms as a unit to obtain additional stroke power, lateral pressure, guidance, and stability

Additional Reinforcements

Index finger on shank:

- Intraoral fulcrum: Left forefinger gently retracts patient's cheek while applying pressure on instrument shank

Cupping hands, index finger on shank:

- Intraoral fulcrum: Both hands in cupped position. Left forefinger gently retracts patient's cheek while positioned on instrument shank for reinforcement. ■

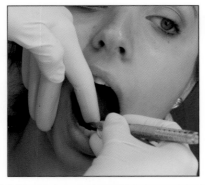

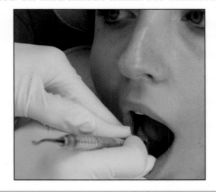

CHAPTER 14

Mandibular Arch, Left Posterior/ Buccal Aspect

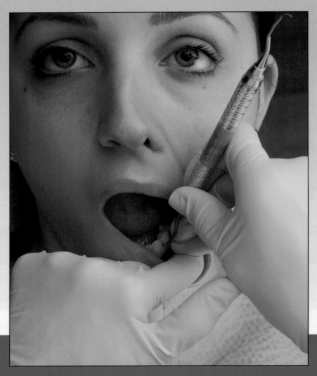

Reinforcement Technique

Conventional Technique

Operator Position:
8:00 - 10:00

Patient Position:
Supine

(Right-handed operator shown)

Buccal Aspect, Mesial Surfaces

- The **Gracey Curet 11/12** is shown

- **Optional instruments:** 5/6 curet for bicuspids, 15/16 curet for molars

- **Working hand:** Intraoral fulcrum stabilized on index finger of reinforcement hand

- **Reinforcement hand:** Left forefinger placed in vestibule while back sides of remaining fingers are supported on patient's jaw

- **Left thumb to right thumb bridging** for reinforcement

- **Technique:** Vertical pull strokes using both hands while utilizing hands and arms as a unit to obtain additional stroke power, lateral pressure, guidance, and stability

Additional Reinforcements

Reinforcement variation:

- Operator position: 1:00 - 2:00

- Extraoral fulcrum: Left forefinger gently retracts patient's cheek

- Left thumb to right thumb bridging

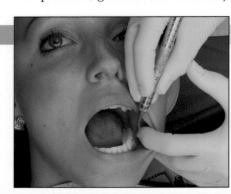

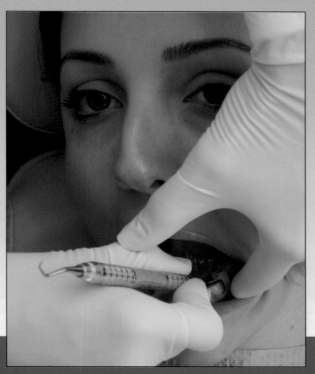

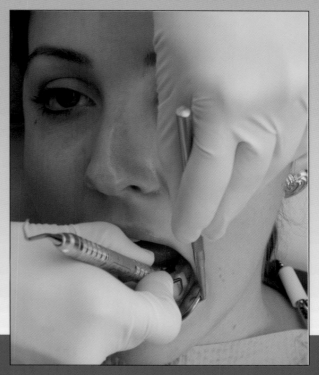

Reinforcement Technique

Conventional Technique

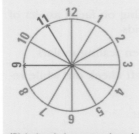

(Right-handed operator shown)

Buccal Aspect, Direct Buccal Surfaces

- The **Gracey Curet 7/8** is shown

- **Optional instrument:** 11/12 curet

- **Working hand:** Extraoral fulcrum with fingers resting on facial aspect of patient's lower anterior teeth and on chin

- **Reinforcement hand:** Left forefinger gently retracts left cheek out while remaining fingers hold on to patient's cheek and jaw

- **Left thumb to right thumb bridging** for reinforcement

- **Technique:** Overlapping diagonal and/or horizontal pull strokes using both hands and arms as a unit to obtain additional stroke power, lateral pressure, guidance, and stability

Additional Reinforcements

Thumb on shank:

- Extraoral fulcrum: Left forefinger gently retracts patient's cheek

- Left thumb on shank or instrument handle applying lateral pressure

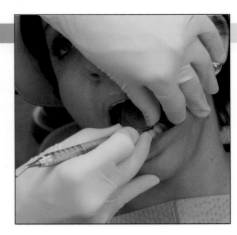

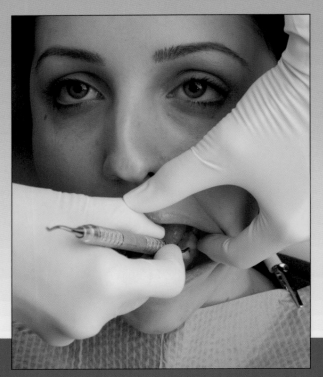

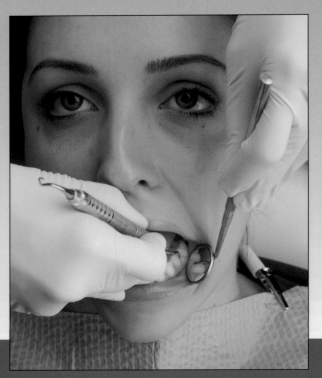

Reinforcement Technique

Conventional Technique

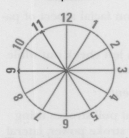
Buccal Aspect, Distal Surfaces

- The **Gracey Curet 13/14** is shown

- **Optional instrument:** 17/18 curet for molars

- **Working hand (a):** Extraoral fulcrum with fingers resting on facial aspect of patient's anterior teeth and chin when scaling bicuspids

- **Working hand (b):** Intraoral fulcrum on bicuspids when scaling molars

- **Reinforcement hand:** Left forefinger gently retracts left cheek out while remaining fingers hold on to patient's cheek and jaw

- **Left thumb to right thumb bridging** for reinforcement

- **Technique:** Vertical pull strokes using both hands and arms as a unit to obtain additional stroke power, lateral pressure, guidance, and stability

Additional Reinforcements

Index finger on shank:

- Extraoral and intraoral fulcrums: Left forefinger gently retracts cheek out while applying pressure on instrument shank

- Left thumb to right thumb bridging for reinforcement ■

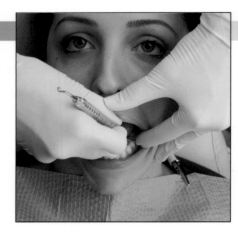

CHAPTER 15

Mandibular Arch, Left Posterior/ Lingual Aspect

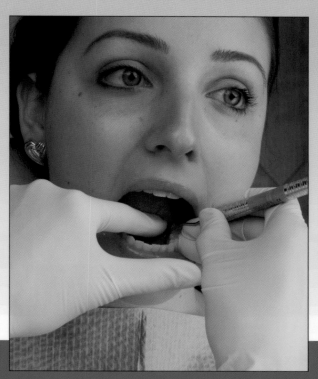

Reinforcement Technique

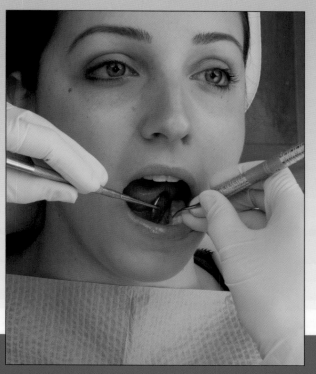

Conventional Technique

Operator Position:
8:00 - 9:00

Patient Position:
Supine

(Right-handed operator shown)

Lingual Aspect, Mesial Surfaces

- The **Gracey Curet 11/12** is shown

- **Optional instruments:** 5/6 curet for bicuspids, 15/16 curet for molars

- **Working hand:** Intraoral fulcrum on mandibular anteriors or bicuspids

- **Reinforcement hand:** Left forefinger gently retracts tongue while back sides of remaining fingers press against patient's cheek and jaw

- **Left thumb to right thumb bridging** for reinforcement

- **Technique:** Vertical pull strokes using both hands while utilizing hands and arms as a unit to obtain additional stroke power, lateral pressure, guidance, and stability

Additional Reinforcements

Reinforcement variation:

- Operator position: 12:00 – 1:00

- Extraoral fulcrum: Left forefinger gently retracts patient's left cheek

- Left thumb to right thumb bridging

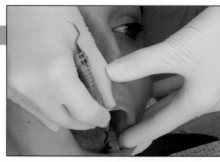

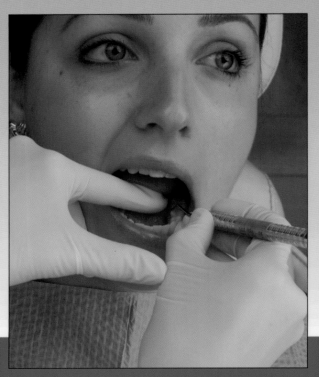

Reinforcement Technique

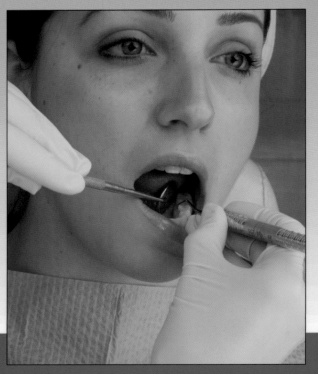

Conventional Technique

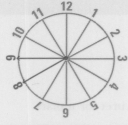

Operator Position:
8:00 - 9:00

Patient Position:
Supine

(Right-handed operator shown)

Lingual Aspect, Direct Lingual Surfaces

- The **Gracey Curet 7/8** is shown

- **Optional instrument:** 11/12 curet

- **Working hand:** Intraoral fulcrum on mandibular anteriors or bicuspids

- **Reinforcement hand:** Left forefinger gently retracts tongue while back sides of remaining fingers press against patient's cheek and jaw

- **Left thumb to right thumb bridging** for reinforcement

- **Technique:** Overlapping diagonal and/or horizontal pull strokes using both hands and arms as a unit to obtain additional stroke power, lateral pressure, guidance, and stability

Additional Reinforcments

Index finger on shank:

- Intraoral fulcrum: Left forefinger guides and presses on instrument handle or shank

- Left thumb to right thumb bridging

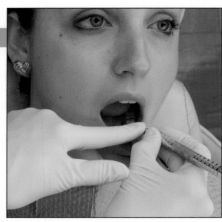

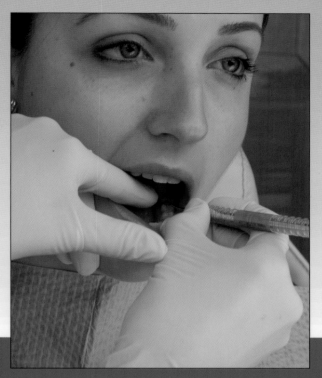

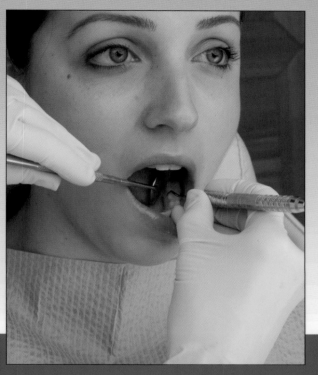

Reinforcement Technique

Conventional Technique

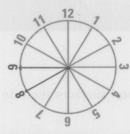

Operator Position:
8:00 - 9:00

Patient Position:
Supine

(Right-handed operator shown)

Lingual Aspect, Distal Surfaces

- The **Gracey Curet 13/14** is shown
- **Optional instrument:** 17/18 curet for molars
- **Working hand:** Intraoral fulcrum on mandibular anteriors or bicuspids
- **Reinforcement hand:** Left forefinger gently retracts tongue while back sides of remaining fingers press against patient's cheek and jaw
- **Left thumb to right thumb bridging** for reinforcement
- **Technique:** Vertical pull strokes using both hands and arms as a unit to obtain additional stroke power, lateral pressure, guidance, and stability

Additional Reinforcements

Index finger on shank:

- Intraoral fulcrum: Both hands are in a cupped position while left forefinger guides and presses on instrument shank
- Left thumb to right thumb bridging ■

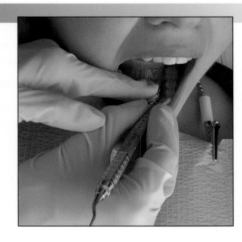

CHAPTER 16

Mandibular Arch, Anterior/Facial Aspect, Mesial And Distal Surfaces

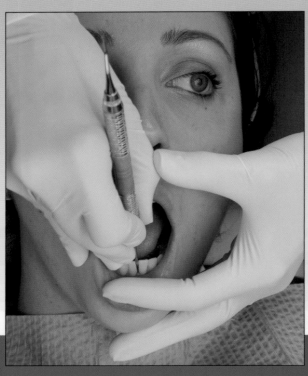

Reinforcement Technique

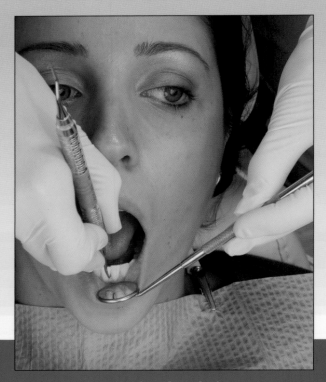

Conventional Technique

Facial Aspect, Mesial and Distal Surfaces

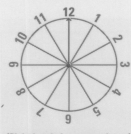

Operator Position:
12:00

Patient Position:
Supine

(Right-handed operator shown)

Note: Mesial surfaces include #25M – #27M and distal surfaces include #22D – #24D.

- The **Gracey Curet 5/6** is shown
- **Optional instruments:** 1/2 and 7/8 curets
- **Working hand:** Intraoral fulcrum on mandibular anterior teeth or bicuspid teeth
- **Reinforcement hand:** Left forefinger gently retracts lower lip while remaining fingers support patient's lower jaw and chin
- **Left thumb to right thumb bridging** for reinforcement
- **Technique:** Vertical pull strokes using both hands and arms as a unit to obtain additional stroke power, lateral pressure, guidance, and stability ■

CHAPTER 17

Mandibular Arch, Anterior/Lingual Aspect, Mesial And Distal Surfaces

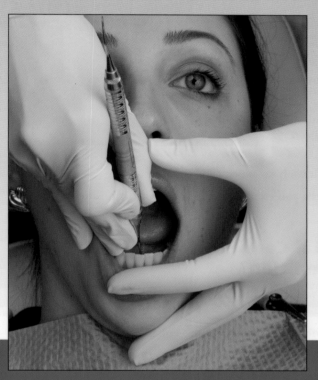

Reinforcement Technique

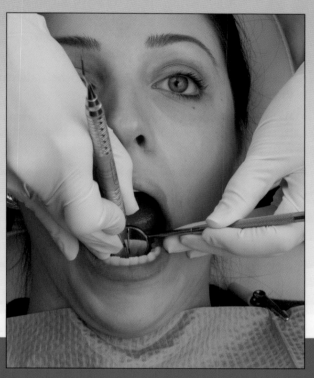

Conventional Technique

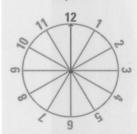

Operator Position:
12:00

Patient Position:
Supine

(Right-handed operator shown)

Lingual Aspect, Mesial and Distal Surfaces

Note: Mesial surfaces include #25M – #27M and distal surfaces include #22D – #24D.

- The **Gracey Curet 5/6** is shown
- **Optional instruments:** 1/2 and 7/8 curets
- **Working hand:** Intraoral fulcrum on mandibular anterior teeth or bicuspid teeth
- **Reinforcement hand:** Left forefinger gently retracts patient's lip while remaining fingers support patient's jaw and chin
- **Left thumb to right thumb bridging** for reinforcement
- **Technique:** Vertical pull strokes using both hands and arms as a unit to obtain additional stroke power, lateral pressure, guidance, and stability

Additional Reinforcments

Thumb on shank:

- Extraoral fulcrum: Left forefinger gently retracts patient's lip
- Left thumb on instrument handle applying lateral pressure ■

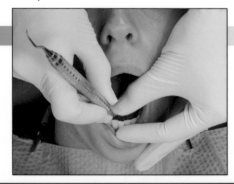

CHAPTER 18

Joint Hyperlaxity

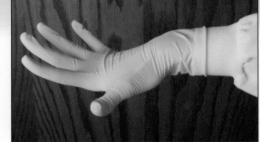

Joint hyperlaxity is a condition where some or all of the joints in the body have an unusually large range of motion, movement, or flexibility.

Causes of Joint Hyperlaxity

- The shape of the ends of the bones (where they move at the joints)

- Weak or stretched ligaments caused by problems with collagen and other proteins (the ligament bands that hold your joints in place)

- Muscle tone (which affects whether joints are held loosely or more rigidly)

- Sense of joint movement (which is the sense that tells you exactly where your joint is positioned and whether it is overstretched)

Why Is It Important for the Dental Care Provider to Recognize a Joint Hyperlaxity Condition?

- Individuals who have flexible joints in their fingers will have difficulty grasping an instrument without having the thumb collapse or hyperextend on the instrument

- Acquiring needed lateral pressure to scale is often difficult when the thumb collapses on the instrument

- Musculoskeletal injuries can occur from extensive force and stress that is applied to the ligaments

What Can Be Done to Minimize Musculoskeletal Injuries that Can Occur from Joint Hyperlaxity?

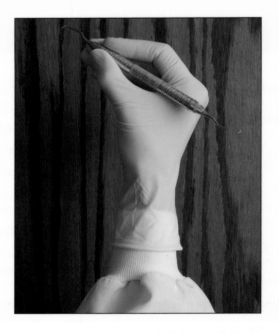

- The dental care provider needs to counter the hyperextension by holding the instrument with a bent thumb, not a collapsed thumb

- The reinforced periodontal instrumentation techniques shown in this manual should be implemented in order to minimize stress and strain on the joints ■

CHAPTER 19

Musculoskeletal Health in Dentistry

Balanced operator posture and optimum ergonomics of the working environment will reduce occupational injuries and ensure career longevity. Musculoskeletal disorders of the back are the leading cause of occupational injury and worker's compensation disability.

Suggestions to obtain musculoskeletal health and optimum performance follow.

Protective Postural Strategies for Optimum Musculoskeletal Health

- Maintain a comfortable neutral posture while working by keeping the shoulders balanced over the hips
- Position operator equipment to allow easy access around the patient
- Keep legs separated and rested on the floor while sitting tall in the chair utilizing magnification
- Modify sitting position throughout the appointment by moving from the 8:00 to 2:00 position
- Keep hips forward toward the operatory chair by using a runner's stance or straddle
- Slightly brace your arm against patient's arm or shoulder for stabilization when additional lateral pressure is needed
- Keep forearms and elbows parallel to the floor and at 30 – 40 degrees as much as possible while scaling to help maintain a relaxed shoulder position
- Minimize hyperextension and hyperflexion of the hand
- Maintain a straight hand-arm-wrist position while using instruments
- Use full arm strokes in place of wrist or finger action when possible in order to use larger arm muscles, which are more powerful and less susceptible to injury
- Stretch your back in the chair during the appointment if discomfort occurs
- Try new postural techniques in order to eradicate bad postural habits
- Utilize an ergonomic chair with adjustable seating height, lumbar support, and forward tilt

Protective Postural Patient Positioning

- Adjust patient's head to allow comfortable positioning while working. Posture is controlled by the patient's head position
- Position patient in supine position to allow control of the angle of patient's maxillary plane
- Promote comfort and relaxation to encourage patient compliance
- Have patient move his or her head to enhance fulcrum position for maximum control and less physical demand
- Use a contoured neck pillow to enhance comfort and compliance when patient has neck problems or limitations
- Have patient tilt his or her head up or down, left or right as needed to assist you
- Have patient adjust mandible minimally or maximally for preferred mouth opening
- Elevate patient up or down in the chair as necessary for appropriate ergonomic positioning technique
- Move patient chair when necessary for around-the-clock operator access and for proper focal distance

Musculoskeletal Injuries Commonly Seen in Dental Care Providers

Carpal Tunnel Syndrome

Carpal tunnel syndrome is a compression or entrapment of the nerves in the wrist. Classic carpal tunnel syndrome is an entrapment of the median nerve, though the radial and ulnar nerves can also be effected. Repetitive flexion and extension of the wrist and hand results in compression of the nerve, primarily the median nerve. Early symptoms include radiating pain, tingling, and numbness in the thumb, index, middle, and ring fingers. Chronic symptoms can progress to include hand weakness, loss of sensation, altered motor skills, and loss of strength.

Ulnar Nerve Neuropathy

Ulnar nerve dysfunction involves impaired movement or sensation in the wrist and forearm. This is caused by injury, entrapment, or compression of the ulnar nerve. The injury or compression can occur as a result of a single event such as a fall or a repetitive injury from continuous or pro-longed flexion and extension of the wrist and forearm. The ulnar nerve travels down the arm from the elbow to the wrist and supplies flexion movement to the wrist and hand. Early symp-toms include pain, tingling, or numbness into the ring and baby fingers. Chronic symptoms may progress to include weakness, loss of strength, and altered motor skills of the involved hand.

Tedonitis

Characterized as an inflammation, irritation, and/or swelling of a tendon, which is a fibrous structure that joins the muscles to the bone. Tendonitis in the wrist and forearm can occur as a result of overuse from repetitive flexion and extension, as well as from poor body mechanics. Symptoms include tenderness along the tendon in proximity to the joint, pain with movement or activity, and loss of strength.

Thoracic Outlet Syndrome

Thoracic outlet syndrome is a condition characterized by pain in the neck and shoulder, numb-ness and tingling of the fingers, and weakening of grip strength of the hand. The syndrome occurs from a compression of the brachial plexus (a bundle of nerves extending from the neck to the shoulder). The compression can be congenital, due to an extra cervical rib, or acquired. Individuals with long necks and droopy shoulders from poor posture may have a greater disposition to this condition. Poor posture, including extending the head and neck in a forward and awkward position with prolonged incorrect postural techniques where shoulders are rounded in a static position, may create pressure on the brachial plexus leading to thoracic outlet syndrome. Symptoms include radiating pain and numbness into the shoulder, arm, wrist, and hand, coupled with weakness and loss of grip strength.

Work-Related Musculoskeletal Injuries of the Spine

Scoliosis

Scoliosis is an abnormal lateral curvature of the spine. It is usually congenital, though it can be acquired from pro-longed lateral or rotated positioning toward the patient. This predisposes the muscles to become shortened on one side of the spine, trigger muscle spasms, and induce chronic pain. Self-induced scoliosis is the body's attempt to adapt to abnormal body position. Early symptoms include chronic one-sided pain, especially in the upper back.

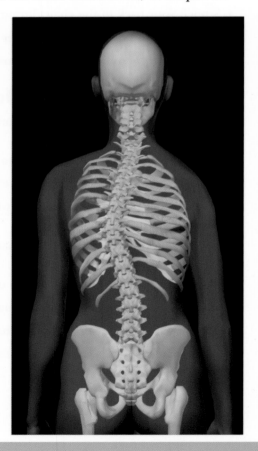

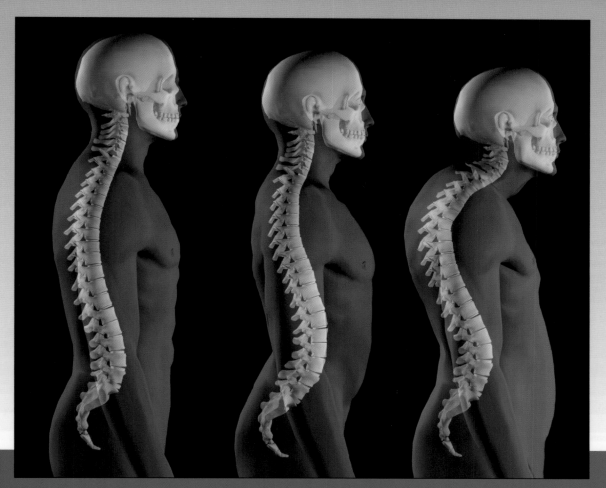

Kyphosis (right) vs. lordosis (middle) vs. normal (left).

Kyphosis

Kyphosis is an abnormal increase in normal kyphotic curvature of the thoracic spine. This can occur as a result of prolonged poor posture, which includes excessive rounding of the shoulders while working on patients. The result is a prominent round back musculoskeletal deformity. Symptoms of increased kyphosis include pain, stiffness, and loss of range of motion.

Increased Lordosis

An increased curvature in the lumbar spine that can be a congenital problem but often is associated with poor posture from prolonged or abnormal positioning. When the lower curve is exaggerated inward, the condition is called lordosis or swayback. The buttocks appear prominent as a result of the excessive arching. Too much of a curve in the low back puts pressure on the entire back. This can lead to increased strain of the lower back that may cause low back pain, sciatica/leg pain, lack of mobility, and disability. ■